The BEST WAYS TO LOOSE WEIGHT FOR UNDER 50

Unlocking the ultimate Guide to Effortless Weight Loss for the 50 and Under Crowd"

By

Rebecca T. Garon

Table of Contents

III. Creating a Calorie Deficit
A. Explanation of calorie deficit
B. Overview of different
methods for creating a calorie
deficit
1. Reducing calorie intake
through diet
2. Increasing physical activity
3. Combination of both
C. Factors to consider when
creating a calorie deficit
1. Health conditions
2. Individual differences
3. Sustainable lifestyle changes

IV. Choosing a Healthy Diet
A. Explanation of the
importance of a healthy diet for
weight loss

B. Overview of macronutrients and micronutrients

C. Tips for building a healthy diet

1. Choosing whole foods

2. Prioritizing protein and fiber

3. Limiting processed foods and added sugars

4. Managing portion sizes

V. Incorporating Physical Activity

A. Explanation of the importance of physical activity for weight loss

B. Overview of different types of physical activity

1. Aerobic exercise

2. Strength training

2. Building support networks
3. Prioritizing self-care
4. Continuing healthy habits

VII. Conclusion
A. Recap of the key points
B. Final thoughts on the importance of healthy weight management for the under 50 population

INTRODUCTION

Most people want to lose weight, but there are so many various diets, exercise regimens, and weight reduction products that it can be confusing to know where to begin. In actuality, altering your lifestyle in a way that is personalized to your unique requirements and goals is the most effective approach to lose weight. We'll look at some of the best weight-loss strategies in this book, including sensible eating practices, consistent exercise, and methods for changing one's behavior. The advice we provide in this article can assist you in achieving your weight reduction objectives in a healthy and long-lasting manner, whether you're trying to lose a few pounds or make a big lifestyle shift.

Chapter 1

Explanation of the importance of maintaining a healthy weight

The key to overall health and wellbeing is to maintain a healthy weight. When someone keeps a healthy weight, it indicates that their body weight is within a range that is thought to be healthy for their height, age, and gender. The usual way to do this is to maintain a balance between the calories you eat and the calories you burn off through exercise and everyday physiological activities.

Keeping a healthy weight is crucial for a number of reasons, some of which are listed below:

Reduces the risk of chronic diseases: Being overweight or obese is a major risk factor for many chronic diseases, including diabetes, heart disease, high blood pressure, stroke, and several types of cancer. The likelihood of contracting these diseases can be lowered by keeping a healthy weight.

Enhances mental health:
Keeping a healthy weight is a way to maintain good mental health. An increased risk of sadness, anxiety, and other mental health conditions has been related to being overweight or obese, according to studies. The mood and general mental health of a person may be enhanced by keeping a healthy weight.

improves physical function:
Being overweight can put stress on the body, making it harder to move around and carry out regular tasks. In order to move more freely and carry out chores more readily, one can

increase physical function by maintaining a healthy weight.

Increasing energy: Being overweight or obese might make you feel tired and low-spirited. A person may feel more energized and more capable of standing for longer if they keep a healthy weight.

Enhances the quality of sleep: Overweight and obesity can have a negative impact on sleep and contribute to diseases like sleep apnea. An individual may be able to enhance their sleep and lower their risk of sleep-related illnesses by keeping a healthy weight.

Overall, it's critical to keep your weight in check if you want to be healthy and happy. Chronic illness risk can be decreased, mental health can be enhanced, physical function can be improved, energy levels can be increased, and sleep quality can be improved. Individuals can reach and maintain a healthy weight, which results in a healthier and happier life, by consuming a balanced diet and exercising on a regular Day.

Chapter 2

Overview of the prevalence of obesity in the under 50 populations

Having an impact on people of all ages, obesity has emerged as a major public health issue worldwide. Obesity has been more prevalent in recent years, especially among people under 50. Having too much body fat raises your risk of developing a number of health issues, which is what is meant by the term "obesity."

The frequency of obesity among people under 50 has

increased to worrying levels in
several nations. This expanding
issue is a result of sedentary
lifestyles, unhealthy diets, and
environmental causes.

Obesity rates appear to be
higher in younger age groups
than in older persons,
according to data from
numerous research and
surveys. The higher prevalence
of obesity among young people
is attributed to factors like poor
eating patterns, rising
processed food consumption,
high sugar intake, and
decreased physical activity.

There are serious health hazards associated with obesity in people under 50. Chronic illnesses like type 2 diabetes, some malignancies, and musculoskeletal issues are more likely to develop as a result. Furthermore, obesity in younger people may have a long-term negative impact on their general health and wellbeing.

It takes a multifaceted approach to combat the prevalence of obesity. It is imperative to encourage active living, regular exercise, and healthy eating habits. To put effective public health measures into place, governments, healthcare providers, and communities must work together. Programs for education, nutritional labeling, encouraging physical exercise in workplaces and schools, and developing surroundings that support healthy living are a few examples of what this might entail.

The prevalence of obesity differs throughout various nations, areas, and communities, and this needs to be noted. Understanding the precise causes of obesity in the population under 50 and developing therapies that take those causes into account require the gathering, monitoring, and analysis of data.

An important public health issue is addressing the prevalence of obesity in the population under 50. The burden of obesity can be lessened, and the health of younger people can be improved, by putting in place comprehensive initiatives and encouraging healthy lifestyles.

Chapter 3

Understanding Weight Loss

By burning off extra body fat or calories that have been stored, weight loss refers to the act of lowering body weight. Healthy dietary practices, regular exercise, and lifestyle adjustments are combined to attain it.

When a person needs energy, their body can draw on the energy that is stored in fat. Overeating causes weight gain because when you eat more calories than your body requires, the extras are stored as fat. On the other side, if you consume fewer calories than your body requires, it will have to burn fat reserves in order to meet its energy needs, which will cause you to lose weight.

Increasing physical activity, eating less calories, or doing both at once can all lead to weight loss. Instead of relying on crash diets or severe exercise routines, a good weight loss plan should entail gradual, lasting changes in eating patterns and physical activity levels.

It is significant to highlight that losing weight can improve general health by lowering the risk of chronic illnesses like diabetes, heart disease, and some types of cancer. Prior to beginning any weight loss program, it is advised to speak with a healthcare provider. Weight loss should, however, be approached in a healthy and balanced manner.

Chapter 4

A. Explanation of calories and energy balance

Two crucial ideas pertaining to the human body's energy consumption and output are calories and energy balance.

Kilocalories (kcal), another name for calories, are a unit of measurement used to express how much energy a serving of food contains. When we eat, our body breaks down the food's macronutrients (carbohydrates, proteins, and fats) and turns them into energy. Each macronutrient's energy content is expressed in calories, with fats having 9 calories per gram compared to 4 for proteins and carbs.

Energy balance is the ratio between the energy we receive from eating and the energy we expend during exercise and other essential metabolic functions like breathing and controlling body temperature. We are said to be in energy balance when the amount of calories we consume equals the number of calories we spend. This implies that we sustain a constant body weight over time.

A positive energy balance, on the other hand, can eventually result in weight increase if we consume more calories than we expend each day. On the other hand, if we have a negative energy balance, we burn more calories than we take in, which over time might result in weight loss.

For general health and well-being, maintaining a good energy balance is crucial. We can achieve and maintain a healthy weight and lower our chance of developing chronic diseases like type 2 diabetes, heart disease, and some malignancies by eating a nutritious, balanced diet that matches our energy needs and exercising on a regular basis.

Chapter 5

Overview of the role of exercise and diet in weight loss

Many people desire to improve their health and general well-being, and one popular objective is weight loss. Weight loss is largely influenced by two important variables: exercise and food. The significance of exercise and diet in weight loss will be covered in this overview.

Exercise:

All weight loss programs must include exercise. Weight loss may result from its assistance with calorie burning and metabolism stimulation. Regular exercise also aids in muscular growth, which may boost the amount of calories burned while at rest.

Exercises like aerobic activity, weightlifting, and high-intensity interval training (HIIT) are just a few of the several forms of exercise that might aid in weight loss. Running, cycling, and swimming are examples of

aerobic activity that can assist
to enhance cardiovascular
health and burn a lot of
calories. While HIIT helps to
burn more calories in a shorter
period of time, strength
training can aid to enhance
metabolism and develop
muscle.

Diet:

A vital component of weight
loss is diet. The amount of
calories consumed can be
decreased and the number of
calories burned can be
increased with a healthy diet,
which can result in weight loss.
While consuming less calories,

a balanced diet that consists of
a range of nutritious foods,
such as fruits, vegetables,
whole grains, lean proteins,
and healthy fats, can help the
body acquire the nutrients it
requires.

By monitoring food intake and choosing healthier options, one efficient weight-loss method is to cut back on calorie intake. This can be achieved by choosing nutrient-dense foods that are lower in calories and minimizing or eliminating processed and high-calorie foods. The consumption of fewer calories and the promotion of weight loss can also be achieved by adhering to a particular diet plan, such as a low-carb or low-fat diet.

Conclusion:

In summary, weight loss depends on both activity and diet. While a nutritious diet and regular exercise can both help you lose weight and give your body the nutrition it needs, exercise helps you burn calories, speed up your metabolism, and develop muscle. The best method for achieving and maintaining weight loss is to combine regular exercise with a healthy diet. Recalling that weight loss is a slow process will help you maintain your efforts over the long run.

Chapter 6

Importance of building healthy habits

For optimal physical and mental health, one must develop good behaviors. The following justifies the significance of creating healthy habits:

Physical Health: Good habits can help your physical health, like regular exercise and a balanced diet. Exercise keeps you at a healthy weight, improves your muscles and bones, and lowers your risk of developing chronic illnesses like diabetes and heart disease. The minerals and energy the body needs to function effectively and keep its general health are provided by a balanced diet.

Healthful behaviors can also help you be more mentally clear. For instance, regular exercise can enhance mood and assist to lessen stress and anxiety. In addition to enhancing mental performance and lowering the risk of cognitive decline, a balanced diet can also aid.

Improved Sleep: Healthy habit formation can lead to better sleep. Exercise encourages deeper sleep and helps to manage sleep patterns. Sleep quality can also be improved by abstaining from stimulants like caffeine and alcohol before bed.

Energy Levels Can Rise: Energy levels can rise as a result of healthy practices. The body gets the resources and energy it needs to function efficiently from a balanced diet and regular exercise. Productivity gains and a general sense of wellbeing may result from this.

Reduction in the Risk of Chronic Diseases: Diabetes, heart disease, and cancer are just a few of the chronic diseases that healthy practices can lower the risk of. Reduced risk of chronic diseases is mostly due to regular exercise, a healthy diet, and quitting smoking.

A higher quality of life can be attained by forming healthy behaviors. A higher quality of life is facilitated by greater physical and mental health, as well as better sleep, energy, and a lower risk of developing chronic diseases.

In conclusion, cultivating healthy habits is crucial for maintaining one's physical and mental well-being, as well as for improving sleep, boosting energy, lowering the risk of chronic diseases, and improving one's general quality of life. You can establish beneficial habits by making minor adjustments to your everyday routine.

Chapter 7

Creating a Calorie Deficit

A vital element of weight loss is establishing a calorie deficit. A calorie deficit, in simple terms, is when you eat fewer calories than your body requires to maintain your weight. Your body will start using fat reserves as energy when you maintain a calorie deficit over time, which will cause weight reduction.

You must understand your daily caloric needs in order to build a calorie deficit. This can be calculated by first taking into account your level of activity throughout the day and then multiplying it by your basal metabolic rate (BMR), which is the amount of energy your body requires to function at rest.

Knowing how many calories you require each day will allow you to modify your intake and produce a calorie deficit. You can accomplish this by eating less calories overall, moving more, or combining the two.

Since one pound of body fat is equal to about 3,500 calories, a deficit of 500–1,000 calories per day can result in a loss of 1-2 pounds of weight every week. To generate a calorie deficit, nevertheless, in a healthy and long-lasting way, it's crucial to keep in mind.

Extreme changes in physical activity levels or calorie intake can have a negative impact on health and are challenging to maintain over the long run. Plan to lose weight gradually and sustainably by aiming for a moderate calorie deficit.

In order to make sure you are
supplying your body with the
nutrients it need when in a
calorie deficit, it is also crucial
to give priority to
nutrient-dense, whole meals.
Concentrating on protein, fiber,
and healthy fats will keep you
feeling full and give you the
energy you need to continue
exercising.

It's crucial to approach weight loss in a healthy and sustainable manner because creating a calorie deficit can be a beneficial tool for the process. You can accomplish your weight loss objectives while still putting your general health and wellness first by calculating your daily caloric needs and gradually changing your diet and level of physical activity.

Chapter 8

A. Explanation of calorie deficit

When your body is in a calorie deficit, it means that it is burning more calories than it is taking in through food and beverages. You can do this by either consuming fewer calories, exercising more, or doing both at once.

It will begin to burn stored fat to make up the difference when you eat less calories than your body requires to maintain your weight. Eventually, this causes weight loss.

Age, gender, weight, height, and activity level are just a few of the variables that will affect how many calories you must cut out of your diet to lose weight. The majority of people are generally thought to be safe and successful with a deficit of 500–1000 calories per day.

You should be aware that a calorie deficit that is too great can be bad for your health. Rapid weight loss can have a significant impact on one's health in various ways, such as by resulting in muscle loss and vitamin deficiencies. By making small, progressive changes to your food and workout regimen, it's crucial to establish a calorie deficit that lasts.

As a result of your body burning more calories than it takes in, you experience a calorie deficit and lose weight. It's critical to establish a calorie deficit that meets your specific demands while being safe and effective.

Chapter 9

Overview of different methods for creating a calorie deficit

Any weight loss or weight management program must include the creation of a calorie deficit. When you eat less calories than your body requires to maintain your weight, it must use the fat reserves in your body as energy, creating a calorie deficit. A calorie deficit can be achieved using a variety of techniques, some of which are covered below:

Changes to Diet: Altering your diet is one of the best strategies to reduce your caloric intake. In order to do this, you might want to cut back on portion sizes and swap out high-calorie items for lower-calorie alternatives. Reduced intake of carbohydrates, fat, or both might also be a part of it.

A calorie deficit can easily be created through exercise. Your calorie deficit grows as a result of increasing your physical activity. Exercises that fall under this category include both strength training and cardiovascular activities like jogging, cycling, or swimming.

A popular strategy for producing a calorie deficit is intermittent fasting. It calls for alternating between eating and fasting, which can assist lower calorie consumption all around.

Low-Calorie Diets: Eating a diet that is low in calories is another strategy to reduce your caloric intake. By consuming less calories overall than what your body requires, you can achieve this. Extremely low-calorie diets can be challenging to maintain, and they might result in dietary deficiencies, so it's crucial to keep that in mind.

Meal Replacement: Meal replacement bars and shakes are meant to take the place of one or more meals throughout the day, offering a low-calorie substitute for regular meals. These items may be a useful approach to reduce your caloric intake, but it's crucial to pick ones that are of good nutritional value and quality.

Behavioral adjustments: Lastly, achieving a calorie deficit can also be accomplished by changing one's behavior.

Examples of such adjustments include lowering stress levels, obtaining enough sleep, and avoiding emotional eating. By making these adjustments, you may encourage a healthy lifestyle and lower your overall calorie intake.

In conclusion, there are numerous approaches to establishing a calorie deficit, and the most effective one will rely on your personal requirements and preferences. To support your general health and wellbeing, it is crucial to pick a strategy that is sustainable and offers enough nourishment.

Chapter 10

Reducing calorie intake through diet

Dietary calorie restriction is a common strategy for weight loss and management. The fundamental idea of this strategy is to consume less calories than you expend, resulting in a calorie deficit that causes weight loss. Despite the fact that it could appear easy, cutting calories calls for meticulous planning and commitment to a balanced diet. Here are some recommendations for lowering calorie intake through diet:

Plan your meals: Making meal preparations in advance will help you stay away from rash choices that can result in overeating. Make sure your meals are well-balanced and contain a lot of fresh produce, whole grains, lean protein, and fruits.

Reduce the size of your portions to help you feel satisfied while ingesting less calories. To aid in portion control, think about utilizing smaller dishes or bowls.

Choose low-calorie foods: By choosing foods that are high in nutrients but low in calories, you can feel full while consuming less calories. Fruits, vegetables, and lean protein sources are all healthy choices.

Eat less of the high-calorie foods that are low in nutrients and high in calories, such as processed foods, sugary drinks, and high-fat snacks.

Utilize calorie-saving cooking techniques: You can eat tasty food while consuming fewer calories by grilling, baking, or steaming your food.

Water can make you feel full and prevent overeating, so

drink enough of it. Aim to consume eight glasses of water a day or more.

Keeping a meal journal or utilizing a calorie-tracking software can help you keep track of your caloric intake and stay on target.

Overall, calorie restriction through food is a successful strategy for weight loss and maintaining a healthy lifestyle. You may cut calories and reach your weight loss goals by preparing your meals in advance, selecting low-calorie foods, and avoiding high-calorie foods.

Chapter 11
Increasing physical activity

One of the best strategies to reduce weight is to increase physical activity, and people under the age of 50 may benefit the most from this strategy. Exercise can improve your general health and lower your chance of developing chronic diseases like heart disease, diabetes, and some types of cancer, in addition to helping you burn calories and lose body fat.

The idea is to choose physical activities that you enjoy and that fit into your lifestyle because there are many different sorts of physical activity that can help you lose weight. The following are some instances of productive physical activity for weight loss:

Exercise your heart: Swimming, cycling, running, and walking are all excellent ways to burn calories and strengthen your heart.

Resistance training: Strength training exercises, including utilizing resistance bands or weights to build muscle, can speed up metabolism and help you burn more calories throughout the day.

High-intensity interval training (HIIT): Studies have indicated that HIIT workouts, which involve brief bursts of intense exercise followed by periods of rest, are helpful for reducing body fat and enhancing general fitness.

A fun and social method to stay active and motivated is to enroll in a group fitness program, such as a dance class or boot camp.

Whatever form of physical activity you decide to engage in, it's critical to gradually increase the intensity and length of your exercises over time in order to achieve the best effects. Increase your weekly workout time progressively as you progress from a moderate to a vigorous level of activity.

In order to reduce weight, it's crucial to concentrate on healthy eating practices in addition to routine exercise. In addition to making you feel full and content, a diet high in fruits, vegetables, whole grains, and lean protein can give your body the nutrients it needs to stay healthy.

You may develop a weight loss plan that is sustainable and successful, helps you reach your objectives, and enhances your general health and wellbeing by incorporating regular physical activity and appropriate eating practices. Always remember to check with your doctor before starting a new workout or nutrition regimen, particularly if you have any underlying medical conditions or worries.

Chapter 12

Combination of both

Combining a healthy diet with regular exercise can be a successful weight loss strategy. While each element may be significant in and of itself, together they can promote long-term weight loss objectives by fostering a sustained and healthy lifestyle change.

The amount of calories you consume each day is determined by your diet, which is why it is so important for weight loss. You must consume

less calories than you burn
each day in order to lose
weight. This can be done by
altering your eating habits,
such as consuming fewer
high-calorie foods and drinks
and eating smaller portions of
healthy foods.

A nutritious diet can give your
body the resources it needs to
function correctly and
encourage physical exercise, in
addition to aiding in weight
loss. For instance, taking
enough carbohydrates can give
you the energy you need to go
through workouts while eating
a diet high in protein can help

you create and maintain
muscle mass.

Exercise is essential for weight
loss since it increases muscle
mass and helps you burn
calories. You burn more
calories when at rest if you
have higher muscle mass,
which can aid in achieving and
maintaining a healthy weight.

Exercise on a regular basis can also assist to enhance mood, energy levels, and cardiovascular health. For best results, try a mix of aerobic and strength training routines. This can include exercises like weightlifting, yoga, running, and cycling.

general, a good diet and consistent exercise can promote your general health and well-being while also assisting you in reaching your weight loss objectives. Instead of concentrating on short-term fixes that might not be sustainable over time, it's crucial to develop sustainable lifestyle adjustments that you can keep up with.

Chapter 13

Factors to consider when creating a calorie deficit

1: Health Conditions: It's important to take into account any existing health conditions you could have before beginning any calorie deficit strategy. Some illnesses, such diabetes, heart disease, or metabolic problems, may call for special dietary considerations or medical supervision. To be sure your weight reduction strategy is secure and suitable for your unique medical requirements, speak with a doctor or qualified nutritionist.

2: Individual Differences:
Because each person is different, variables including age, sex, weight, height, body composition, and degree of activity can have a big impact on calorie needs. It's critical to tailor your calorie deficit to your unique requirements and objectives. Determine a reasonable calorie deficit for you by calculating your basal metabolic rate (BMR) and total daily energy expenditure (TDEE). It's generally advised to lose weight gradually and sustainably, aiming for a daily

caloric deficit of 500–1000 calories to lose roughly 1-2 pounds each week.

3: Sustainable Lifestyle: It's important to design a calorie deficit strategy that works well with your way of life and is long-lasting. In general, crash diets and highly restricted methods are unsustainable and can result in dietary deficits, muscle loss, and a higher chance of gaining weight again. Choose a well-rounded strategy that emphasizes portion control, emphasizes a range of nutrient-dense foods, and promotes healthy routines like frequent exercise.

Chapter 14

Choosing a Healthy Diet and Explanation of the importance of a healthy diet for weight loss

For a number of reasons, a nutritious diet is vital for losing weight. To lose weight, you need to eat less calories than you burn off each day, which is known as creating a calorie deficit. But just as essential as how much food you eat is the quality of it. The significance of a good diet for weight loss is explained in the following ways:

Calorie Control: A nutritious diet emphasizes items low in calories but high in nutrients, such as fruits, vegetables, whole grains, and lean proteins. These foods typically include vital nutrients, vitamins, and minerals while also being more full and satisfying the appetite. These choices allow you to eat more food for less calories while still feeling full, which can help you reach a calorie deficit.

Nutritional Balance: With a diet that is well-balanced, you can be confident that your body is getting all the nutrients it needs for optimum performance.
Making every calorie count by consuming nutrient-dense foods becomes even more important as your caloric intake decreases. Muscle maintenance, satiety, and long-lasting energy are supported by an adequate protein, healthy fats, and complex carbohydrate intake.

Maintaining overall health while losing weight is supported by proper diet, which helps prevent vitamin deficits.

Weight reduction That Is Sustainable: Although severe weight reduction techniques like crash diets or abstinence only plans can cause initial weight loss that is quick, they are frequently not long-term solutions. Such diets frequently lack critical nutrients, which may result in muscle loss, a slowed metabolism, and detrimental impacts on general health. You can nourish your body while gradually losing

weight by choosing a balanced
diet.

The process by which your
body transforms food into
energy, known as metabolism,
can be favourably impacted by
eating a balanced diet. Your
metabolism typically runs at
peak efficiency when you
regularly eat nutrient-dense
foods. Even while at rest, this
can increase your ability to
burn calories. In contrast,
eating a lot of processed food,
sweet treats, and fat might slow
down your metabolism and
make it harder to lose weight.

Changes in behavior: A nutritious diet promotes conscious eating and the formation of healthy eating habits. You may train yourself to be more aware of your body's hunger and fullness cues by selecting healthful foods and paying attention to portion choices. As a result, weight control is improved by preventing overeating and emotional eating.

Benefits to Overall Health: Losing weight with a balanced diet has several advantages to overall health in addition to helping you lose weight. Chronic illnesses like high blood pressure, type 2 diabetes, cancer, and heart disease can all be decreased by it. Optimal organ function, hormone balance, and general wellbeing are supported by feeding your body the correct nutrients.

The key to efficient and long-lasting weight loss is a nutritious diet, in conclusion. It offers extra health advantages in addition to providing the required nutrients, aiding with calorie restriction, supporting metabolism, and promoting long-term behavior change.

You can reach your weight loss objectives while upholding optimum health by exercising moderation in your food choices and following a balanced diet.

Chapter 15

B. Overview of macronutrients and micronutrients

Macronutrients:

The body uses carbohydrates as its main energy source. They are present in foods like cereals, fruits, vegetables, legumes, and legume products. Simple carbohydrates (like sugars) and complex carbohydrates (such starches and fibre) are two different types of carbohydrates.

Proteins: Proteins are necessary for the development, maintenance, and repair of all bodily tissues. They are composed of amino acids and can be obtained from foods such as meat, fish, poultry, dairy products, legumes, and nuts. Additionally, proteins are involved in the creation of hormones and enzymatic processes.

Fats: Fats are concentrated energy sources that are essential for sustaining cell structure, insulating organs, and controlling body temperature. They can be found in foods like oils, butter, nuts, seeds, and fatty meats. Unsaturated fats are generally seen as being healthier than saturated and trans fats.

Micronutrients:

Vitamins: Vitamins are organic substances that the body needs in little amounts for a variety of metabolic processes. They are divided into two categories: fat-soluble vitamins (such vitamins A, D, E, and K) and water-soluble vitamins (like vitamins C and the B-complex). Each vitamin supports particular biological activities in a distinct way and can be obtained through a balanced diet.

Minerals: Minerals are inorganic substances that are necessary in minute amounts for a variety of physiological activities. They comprise both macrominerals like calcium, phosphorus, magnesium, sodium, and potassium as well as trace minerals like iron, zinc, iodine, copper, and selenium. Minerals are essential for maintaining healthy bones, nerves, fluid balance, and enzyme functions.

For sustaining general health and wellbeing, both

macronutrients and micronutrients are essential. Micronutrients are important in controlling multiple biochemical events and supporting diverse physiological functions, whereas macronutrients give the body energy and structural components. To meet the body's nutritional requirements, it's crucial to eat a balanced diet that contains enough macronutrients and micronutrients.

Chapter 16

Advice on creating a healthy diet

Making thoughtful food selections is a necessary component of creating a balanced diet. The following advice will assist you in developing a wholesome and well-balanced diet:

1. Choosing whole foods: Whole foods are minimally processed and include all the nutrients that are present in them naturally. Fruits, vegetables, whole grains, lean proteins, and healthy fats are among them. These foods offer necessary vitamins, minerals, and dietary fiber and are typically more nutrient-dense.

2. Giving protein and fiber the highest priority: A healthy diet should prioritize both of these nutrients. Building and mending tissues, boosting the immune system, and preserving lean muscle mass all depend on protein. Lean meats, poultry, fish, eggs, legumes, nuts, and seeds are all good sources of protein. Fiber facilitates digestion, encourages feelings of fullness, and helps control blood sugar levels. Dietary fiber is

abundant in whole grains,
fruits, vegetables, legumes,
nuts, and whole grains.

**3: Limiting additional sugars
and processed foods:** Processed
foods frequently contain large
amounts of harmful fats,
sodium, and added sugars.
These foods have little
nutritional value and only
provide empty calories.
Instead, concentrate on eating
as many fresh, unadulterated
meals as you can. Added sugars
should also be avoided because
they can lead to weight gain
and other health problems.
Read the labels on your food
and choose naturally sweet

items like fruits or foods with
no added sugar.

4. Managing portion sizes:
Portion control is essential for
keeping a healthy weight and
avoiding overeating. It's
beneficial to pay attention to
portion sizes and your body's
signals of hunger and fullness.
Include a variety of foods from
various dietary categories in
your meals, and work to
balance your plate with the
right amounts of veggies,
grains, and proteins. To make
sure you're satisfying your
nutritional needs without
consuming too many calories,

stay away from huge quantities and eat in moderation.

Always keep in mind that developing a healthy diet is not about following strict rules or depriving yourself of particular items. It involves making enduring, well-balanced decisions that nourish your body and promote overall wellbeing. Working with a licensed dietitian can help you create a nutrition plan that is customised for your requirements and goals.

Chapter 17

Incorporating Physical Activity

Your entire health and well-being can be enhanced by include physical activity in your everyday routine. There are many ways to incorporate physical activity into your life, whether your goal is to reduce weight, improve your fitness level, or simply enjoy the many advantages of exercise. To get you started, consider the following ideas:

Exercise plan for the morning: To jump-start your metabolism and give yourself energy, start your day with a quick workout. Bodyweight exercises, yoga, or a brisk walk or jog around your neighborhood are all simple workouts you can complete at home.

Active Commute: If at all possible, choose to bike or walk to work rather than to drive or take public transportation. This enables you to include physical activity in your everyday routine and lessens your carbon footprint, which benefits the environment.

Take Active Breaks: Instead than spending the entire day seated at a desk, get up from your chair and stretch for a few minutes. To get your blood circulating and increase your energy levels, try easy activities like squats, lunges, or push-ups.

Walks during Lunch: Take advantage of your break during lunch to go for a quick stroll. Find a park or other area of greenery in the neighborhood so you can get some fresh air and exercise. Walking has health advantages for both your body and mind, and it increases productivity.

Elevator or Stairs? Whenever possible, take the stairs. Engaging your leg muscles and raising your heart rate can be accomplished by climbing steps.

Active Hobbies: Look for pursuits or pastimes that call for mobility. Get involved in a sports league, learn to dance, or attend a martial arts session. Exercise will become less of a chore and more of an enjoyable activity if you engage in things you enjoy.

Activities with Family or Friends: Get your family and

friends involved in physical activity. Take a group out for a bike ride, play some soccer, or plan weekend hiking. You'll be encouraging each other to be active while also spending time with your loved ones.

Look into online fitness courses or exercise applications that match your hobbies and fitness level. There are several options available that may be done from the comfort of your own home, ranging from yoga sessions to high-intensity workouts.

Spending your leisure time actively will keep you more

active than sitting in front of
the TV or computer. Play
outdoor games like frisbee,
have a swim, or go biking
around your neighborhood.

Track Your Progress: Keep
track of how much you exercise
each day with a fitness tracker
or a smartphone app. You can
stay motivated and dedicated
to your exercise regimen by
setting objectives and
monitoring your progress.

Chapter 18

Explanation of the importance of physical activity for weight loss

For a variety of reasons, physical activity is essential for weight loss. Incorporating regular exercise into your routine will considerably increase the effectiveness of your weight loss attempts, even though nutrition is an important aspect in weight management. Here are several main justifications for why physical exercise is essential for weight loss:

Caloric Expenditure: Physical exercise boosts your body's calorie expenditure. Your body needs energy to carry out movements when you exercise, whether you're walking, jogging, cycling, or doing weight training. The calories that are kept in your body as fat reserves and other forms of storage provide this energy. You can lose weight by creating an energy deficit by continually burning more calories than you take in.

Lean muscle mass development is encouraged by exercise, which also helps to maintain it. Muscle tissue

burns more calories at rest
than fat tissue because it has a
higher metabolic activity. Your
metabolism is stimulated as
you gain muscle through
workouts like strength training,
which causes an increase in
calorie burn even when you're
not actively exercising. This
may aid in sustained weight
loss and weight management.

Exercise on a regular basis can
assist control and enhance your
metabolic rate. Exercise
increases the release and
production of several
hormones, including growth
hormone and adrenaline,
which can boost metabolic

activity. Weight reduction results from your body using stored fat and other forms of energy more effectively when your metabolism is optimized.

Appetite Control: Exercise has the power to alter your appetite and improve how you regulate your food intake. By changing some hunger-related chemicals, intense workouts, especially cardiovascular ones, might temporarily lower appetite. Regular exercise has also been demonstrated to increase the sensitivity of hormones that control hunger, including leptin and ghrelin, making it simpler to maintain a good calorie balance and lessen overeating.

Numerous psychological advantages of physical activity assist with weight loss attempts in an indirect manner. Endorphins, a class of neurotransmitters released during exercise, help to promote sensations of enjoyment and wellbeing. Regular exercise can ease the tension, anxiety, and despair that are frequently accompanied by emotional eating and weight increase. Exercise can help you achieve a happy mood and retain motivation for weight loss by enhancing your mental health.

Long-Term Weight Maintenance: Physical activity is essential for long-term weight maintenance as well as early weight loss. You develop healthy habits that help you maintain your weight by include regular exercise in your lifestyle. By maintaining muscular mass, promoting metabolic health, and giving them a way to manage stress and their emotions, it helps people avoid gaining weight.

It's crucial to remember that while exercise is essential for weight loss, for best results, it should be accompanied with a healthy, balanced diet. You can create a customized workout program that fits your goals, level of fitness, and any underlying health concerns you might have by speaking with a healthcare provider or a certified fitness expert

Chapter 19

Overview of different types of physical activity

A wide range of motions and exercises are included in physical activity, both of which promote general health and fitness. It is essential for keeping a healthy lifestyle and is divided into several varieties according to its features and advantages. The various forms of physical activity are described below:

Exercise that is aerobic and cardiovascular: Aerobic activities speed up the heart and breathing rates, which benefits the cardiovascular system. Exercises that fit into this category include jogging, running, swimming, cycling, dancing, and brisk walking. They bolster the heart and lungs while enhancing endurance and burning calories.

Resistance training, often known as strength training, is a technique for working and strengthening muscles by using resistance, such as weights or resistance bands. Bone density is raised, overall strength is improved, and muscular mass is developed. Strength training includes activities like lifting weights, push-ups, squats, and lunges.

Exercises that improve flexibility work to increase muscle elasticity and joint movement. Common methods of increasing flexibility include stretching exercises, yoga, and Pilates. Improved posture, injury prevention, and range of motion are all benefits of these exercises.

Exercises that increase coordination, proprioception, and overall balance are uknown as balance and stability exercises. When it comes to preventing falls, they are especially helpful for elderly persons. Tai chi, yoga, particular balance training drills, and the use of balance boards or stability balls are a few examples.

High-Intensity Interval Training (HIIT): HIIT entails brief bursts of vigorous exercise followed by rest intervals or lower-intensity exercise. In addition to boosting metabolism, it also helps burn calories and increase cardiovascular fitness. High-intensity interval training (HIIT) includes exercises including sprinting, circuit training, and Tabata.

Sports and Recreational Activities: Taking part in sports and recreational activities is a fun way to keep active. Along with the thrill of competition and teamwork, sports like volleyball, basketball, tennis, and soccer provide both cardiovascular and strength advantages.

Outdoor activities: wide variety of physical pursuits that take place in the outdoors are included in the category of outdoor activities. Ones that come to mind are skiing, riding, swimming, and hiking. Exercise, fresh air, and a chance to interact with nature are all benefits of participating in these activities.

Low-impact workouts are mild on the joints and suited for anyone with joint pain or injuries. Low-impact exercises that are good for the heart while being easier on the joints include walking, cycling, swimming, water aerobics, and using elliptical machines.

Improve the movements and strength needed for daily activities through functional training. Lifting, carrying, pushing, and tugging are just a few of the workouts that replicate real-life motions. In addition to improving overall fitness, functional training can also aid in reducing daily injury risk.

A healthcare practitioner or fitness specialist should always be consulted before beginning any new workout regimen, especially if you have any current medical ailments or concerns. On the basis of your unique requirements and objectives, they may offer you individualized advice and direction.

Chapter 20

Tips for incorporating physical activity into daily life.

A healthy lifestyle requires regular physical activity. The following advice will assist you in incorporating exercise into your daily routine:

Start out slowly: Set achievable goals to start, then progressively up your activity level. You might begin with quick strolls or easy activities and gradually increase your endurance and intensity.

Make time for exercise: Consider your everyday workouts to be crucial appointments. Set aside time each day for exercise and keep to it. The key is consistency.

Find activities you like to do: Find physical activities that you actually enjoy doing. Find an activity that makes you happy, whether it be dancing, swimming, cycling, hiking, or participating in a sport. You're more likely to persevere if you appreciate what you're doing.

Include movement breaks:
Move your body briefly during the day. Go take a brief walk, stand up and stretch, or perform some exercises at your desk. These breaks might help you break up times of inactivity and keep you feeling motivated.

Exercise with friends, family, or enroll in a group fitness class to make it a social activity. It will not only make the action more fun, but it will also provide you accountability and drive.

Utilize your surroundings by looking for chances to be active in your regular setting. Use the stairs instead of the elevator, travel by foot or bicycle to nearby destinations, or engage in physically demanding home tasks.

Realistic goals should be specific and doable. It can be increasing your strength in a certain exercise, jogging a specific distance, or taking a certain amount of steps each day. You can maintain motivation by tracking your progress.

Mix it up: Change up your workouts to avoid getting bored. Include a variety of workouts to target various muscle regions while maintaining interest. Additionally, it helps avoid plateaus and overuse injuries.

Make it a family affair by getting everyone moving. Together, go for walks, play sports, or start a new hobby. It's a fantastic method to prioritize exercise while also having quality time.

Find methods to keep inspired as you progress in your fitness. Create incentives for reaching your objectives, monitor your advancement, locate a workout partner, or use technology and fitness applications to keep yourself motivated.

Chapter 21

Maintaining Long-Term Success.

Even though maintaining long-term success with weight loss can be difficult, it is possible to reach and maintain your goal weight with the appropriate tactics and attitude. You may sustain your weight loss achievement by following the following basic principles:

Set Achievable Objectives: Setting achievable objectives is crucial for long-term success. To lose weight, don't set unrealistic or drastic goals. Intend to lose 1-2 pounds consistently and healthily each week. The likelihood of regaining weight is lower with this strategy and it is more maintainable.

Adopt Healthy Eating Habits: Put your attention toward making sure that your daily routine includes nutritious, balanced meals. Embrace a range of fresh produce, nutritious grains, lean proteins, and healthy fats. Sugary drinks, processed foods, and frequent snacking should all be avoided or limited. To avoid overeating, exercise portion control.

Regular Exercise: Exercise regularly to keep off the weight you've lost and to enhance your general health. Set a weekly goal of 75 minutes of strenuous exercise or 150 minutes of moderate aerobic activity. Strength training routines can help you maintain your weight by boosting your metabolism and helping you gain muscle.

Track Your Progress: Keep tabs on your dietary intake, workout schedule, and advancement toward your objectives. You can stay on track with your weight loss goals by keeping a record of your progress and identifying patterns. To keep track of your meals and activities, think about utilizing a mobile app or a food diary.

Use mindful eating to your advantage by paying attention to your body's signals of hunger and fullness. When you feel pleasantly full, stop eating after taking a few deliberate, leisurely bites. Avoid emotional eating by adopting other coping mechanisms to deal with stress or unpleasant feelings, such as taking up a hobby, chatting to a friend, or using relaxation techniques.

Create a Support Network:
Surround yourself with a group of people who will encourage you, such as family, friends, or a weight loss support group. A crucial source of accountability and motivation is having individuals who support your aims. With them, you can discuss your achievements and difficulties and, if necessary, enlist their assistance.

Water is your best hydration source, so sip on it frequently. Digestion can be aided by water, which can also boost general health and help you manage your hunger. Limit your intake of alcohol and sweetened beverages because both can cause you to gain weight.

Be mindful of your stress levels because they can hinder your attempts to lose weight. Find healthy coping mechanisms for stress, such mindfulness, yoga, meditation, or participating in activities you like to do physically. Prioritize obtaining adequate restorative sleep each night since it's essential for stress management and maintaining a healthy weight.

Be Patient With Yourself: Keep in mind that losing weight is a process that may involve setbacks. Don't punish yourself too harshly if you make a mistake or gain a few pounds. Instead, take what you can from the situation, adjust as required, and commit once more to your healthy routines. Instead than focusing on perfection, consider progress.

Regular checkup: Make an appointment for routine checkups with your healthcare provider to assess your general health and go over any worries or difficulties you may be experiencing. They can help you stay on track with your weight reduction and maintenance goals by offering direction, advice, and support that is specifically customized to your needs.

Keep in mind that rather than depending on temporary fixes, maintaining long-term weight loss demands a commitment to a healthy lifestyle. You can improve your chances of maintaining long-term weight loss success by implementing these ideas into your everyday practice.

chapter 22

Explanation of the challenges of maintaining weight loose

Due to a variety of causes, many people may find it difficult to maintain weight loss. The following are some of the typical difficulties people run into when attempting to keep off their weight loss:

Metabolic Adaptation: Your body may slow down as a result of losing weight as a result of consuming less calories.

Because of your body's improved ability to store calories, this metabolic adaptation makes it simpler to acquire weight. Due to this, maintaining weight loss may be more difficult for you if you don't make other dietary and activity regimen changes.

Emotional and psychological elements of weight control can be difficult because weight loss efforts frequently necessitate major lifestyle adjustments. A lot of people battle food cravings, emotional eating, stress, and body image concerns, which can result in overeating and weight gain.

Maintaining weight loss requires a long-term behavioral shift and the creation of a healthy connection with food and one's body.

Unfriendly Environment: A person's surroundings, both socially and environmentally, can have a big impact on their ability to maintain their weight. Maintaining motivation can be challenging when there is a lack of support from loved ones, friends, or coworkers who do not comprehend the difficulties associated with weight management. Additionally, it might be difficult to maintain a healthy weight when you live or work in an atmosphere that encourages sedentary or bad eating habits.

After a first round of weight loss, it's usual to hit a weight plateau or see swings in weight. These times can be discouraging and demoralizing, which might cause some people to fall back on old routines. Keep in mind that swings are common and that weight loss is not always linear. It is essential to continually maintain a healthy lifestyle despite brief setbacks.

Lifestyle Modifications and Sustainability: In order to lose weight successfully, one must frequently make numerous lifestyle adjustments, such as food adjustments, greater physical activity, and improved stress management. On the other hand, it can be difficult to preserve these modifications over time. It can be challenging to maintain the same degree of drive and commitment over time, particularly if the changes feel constrictive or stressful. The secret to lasting weight control is striking a balance between a healthy lifestyle and individual tastes.

Unrealistic Expectations:
Having unattainable
expectations for weight loss
might leave you feeling
disappointed and make it
harder to keep the weight off in
the long run. Many people
think that keeping a set weight
may be easily accomplished,
but in reality, it takes ongoing
effort, commitment, and
adjustment. By realizing that
maintaining a healthy weight is
a lifelong struggle and by
placing more emphasis on
overall health and wellbeing
than just the weight, it is able
to effectively manage
expectations.

Challenges and life Transition: Transitional life events like a job shift, a breakup, or the birth of a child can disrupt patterns and make it more difficult to keep a healthy weight. Stress, a lack of time, or emotional turbulence may lead people to prioritize other aspects of their lives during these transitions over good activities. It is crucial to build resilience and adaptation in order to get beyond these challenges while keeping weight management in mind.

To get beyond these challenges, a dependable weight maintenance plan must be developed. This requires setting realistic goals, asking family, friends, or professionals for help, developing a positive relationship with food, putting emotional eating control skills into practice, and maintaining a regular exercise routine. It's important to remember that maintaining weight loss requires ongoing effort and a lifetime commitment, but it is doable with the right mindset and methods.

chapter 23

Overview of strategies for maintaining weight loss

The long-term maintenance of weight loss might be difficult, but there are a number of tactics that can assist you. Listed below is a summary of a few potent tactics:

Progress tracking: Keeping weight off requires regular weight monitoring and progress tracking. Regular self-weighing is one way to achieve this, as is using other techniques like recording waist circumference or calculating body fat percentage. Maintaining a record of your progress will allow you to see any changes or trends early on and take appropriate action as necessary.

Creating support systems: One of the best ways to keep off weight loss is to surround yourself with a network of people who are willing to help you, whether they be friends, family, or members of your community. Encouragement, inspiration, and accountability can all be obtained from these people. You may keep on track and exchange experiences and advice with others who share your goals by joining weight loss support groups, online communities, or finding a workout partner.

Putting your own needs first: Maintaining weight reduction requires prioritizing your physical, mental, and emotional well-being. Don't forget to give sleep a high priority, to control your tension, and to partake in enjoyable and relaxing activities. Emotional eating and using food as consolation can be avoided by implementing stress management practices like meditation, yoga, or hobby-based activities.

Maintaining healthy behaviors: Keeping up the good habits that got you there is one of the most crucial things you can do to sustain your weight loss. This entails keeping up with healthy lifestyle practices, such as eating a balanced diet that is rich in nutrients, and engaging in frequent physical activity.

Constantly strive to eat a
variety of whole foods, such as
fruits, vegetables, lean
proteins, and whole grains.
Make sure to stay physically
active by partaking in activities
you enjoy, such walking,
jogging, cycling, or strength
training.

Becoming conscious of your eating patterns and portion sizes is also crucial. Refrain from reverting to previous eating behaviors such as bingeing or relying heavily on harmful foods. Instead, seek moderation and a healthy balance that suits you.

It's important to keep in mind that maintaining weight loss is a lifelong process, and variations are to be expected. Accept the journey, practice self-compassion, and honor your successes.

chapter 24
Conclusion

The book "The Best Way to Lose Weight for Under 50" gives a thorough and helpful manual for anyone looking to lose weight on a tight budget. This book is an invaluable resource for anyone trying to reduce weight without going bankrupt because the author consistently offers sage advice, research-supported tactics, and doable actions.

This book's emphasis on adhering to a thorough weight-loss strategy is one of its main advantages. The author advises readers to adopt long-lasting lifestyle adjustments that will assist long-term success rather than promoting fad diets or fast cures. The book gives readers the tools they need to have a positive and rewarding relationship with food by emphasizing the concepts of a balanced diet, portion control, regular exercise, and mindful eating.

Furthermore, "The Best Way to Lose Weight for Under 50" recognizes the financial difficulties that many people have when attempting to lose weight. The author provides readers with useful advice and budget-friendly meal ideas that may aid them in making wise decisions when grocery shopping and dining out. The book provides examples of inexpensive substitutes, accessible forms of exercise, and straightforward yet effective at-home workouts to show that weight loss is feasible for everyone, regardless of their financial position.

This work's evidence-based technique is another noteworthy feature. The author supports their recommendations with expert judgment and scientific research, guaranteeing that the readers are given accurate and trustworthy information. The book dispels common weight loss myths and misconceptions, giving readers the information they need to make knowledgeable decisions about their health.

People who want to start losing weight without going over their budget might find "The Best Way to Lose Weight for Under 50" to be generally beneficial. The book's comprehensive approach, cost-effective methods, and evidence-based suggestions give readers the information and resources they need to lose weight in a healthy, sustainable way. Readers can improve their health, boost their self-esteem, and live full, active lives without breaking the bank by heeding the recommendations offered in this book.

Chapter 25

Recap of the key points

Description: A recap of "The Best Way to Lose Weight for Under 50"

An authoritative manual on weight loss called "The Best Way to Lose Weight for Under 50" was produced by a specialist in the subject and focuses on practical methods designed especially for people under 50. Following is a summary of the book's major themes:

Understanding Weight Loss:
The book begins by outlining
the underlying ideas behind
weight loss, such as the idea of
a calorie deficit, metabolism,
and the significance of forming
enduring habits.

Nutrition: The importance of
eating a balanced, nutritious
diet is heavily stressed. The
book offers information on
portion control, the function of
macronutrients
(carbohydrates, proteins, and
fats), and the significance of
eating whole foods and
avoiding processed and sugary
foods.

Meal Planning: In order to reach weight loss objectives, the author highlights the significance of meal planning. In order to prevent impulsive eating decisions, it provides helpful advice on grocery shopping, planning healthy meals, and cooking ahead of time.

Exercise and physical activity are heavily emphasized in the book as important components of a weight loss program. It highlights a variety of exercises acceptable for people under 50, such as cardio, weight training, and flexibility exercises, while emphasizing the significance of choosing activities that you enjoy and can stick with.

Changes to Your Lifestyle: The author acknowledges the influence of lifestyle variables on weight loss and offers advice on mindful eating, stress reduction, and sleep hygiene. The significance of self-care is emphasized, and potential problems with time management and work-life balance that may be encountered by people under 50 are also discussed.

Progress tracking is crucial for encouraging behavior and holding people accountable.

The book offers numerous strategies for maintaining tabs on weight, physical characteristics, and general health, including the use of apps, journaling, and seeing a specialist.

Overcoming Obstacles and Plateaus: The author understands that obstacles and plateaus may arise over the course of weight loss efforts. The book includes useful guidance on overcoming plateaus, coping with cravings, keeping motivation high, and getting help from others or experts.

The shift from weight loss to weight maintenance is the subject of the book's final part, which is also its most comprehensive. In order to succeed over the long term, it highlights the significance of creating a sustainable lifestyle, establishing attainable goals, and forming wholesome habits.

For anyone looking for individualized weight loss plans that are efficient and long-lasting, "The Best Way to Lose Weight for Under 50" is a great resource. This book gives readers the skills they need to achieve their weight loss objectives and enhance their general well-being by offering helpful guidance on nutrition, exercise, lifestyle adjustments, and long-term maintenance.

Chapter 26

Final thoughts on the importance of healthy weight management for the under 50 population

Keeping a healthy weight is important for people of all ages, but it is especially important for people under the age of 50. Developing and maintaining healthy behaviors during this period of life is crucial for laying the foundation for long-term wellbeing. It is impossible to exaggerate the significance of

good weight management
because it has an impact on
many facets of a person's life,
including physical health,
mental health, and general
quality of life.

In the first place, maintaining a
healthy weight greatly lowers
the risk of contracting many
chronic illnesses. Obesity is
frequently linked to diseases
like heart disease, type 2
diabetes, high blood pressure,
some types of cancer, and joint
issues. People can reduce these
risks by using a healthy weight
management strategy, which
will benefit their long-term
health.

Additionally, maintaining a healthy weight has a good impact on mental health. The population under 50 is frequently focused on demanding careers, starting families, or going to college.

These obligations may result in higher stress levels and a greater risk of developing anxiety and depression. A balanced diet and routine physical activity have repeatedly been proved to reduce stress and enhance mental health. People are more likely to enjoy greater mood, more energy, and more self-esteem when they maintain a healthy weight.

In order to improve quality of life, good weight management is also essential. Achieving and maintaining a healthy weight makes it easier for people to engage in physical activity, which is crucial for those who have families or lead active lifestyles. People are better able to engage in leisure pursuits, pursue hobbies, and enjoy time with loved ones when they maintain a healthy weight. A healthy weight also fosters a favorable relationship with one's own body and has a positive effect on one's self-image and body confidence.

It's crucial to take a healthy, long-term approach to weight management. In addition to being short-term ineffectual, crash diets, intense exercise programs, and inappropriate weight loss techniques can be harmful to both physical and emotional health. Instead, obtaining and maintaining a healthy weight requires a holistic strategy that incorporates consistent exercise, a well-balanced diet, and mindful eating practices. On the path to a healthy weight, consulting with medical experts like registered dietitians or fitness trainers can offer individualized advice and support.

In conclusion, it is crucial for those under 50 to manage their weight in a healthy way. People can lower their chance of developing chronic diseases, boost their mental health, and improve their general quality of life by keeping a healthy weight. Adopting a healthy and sustainable weight-management strategy is essential for long-term success and wellbeing. An individual can build the foundation for a happier and more happy life by giving healthy weight management priority.